Mood Therapy: Cure Your Mood Swings with DBT Exercises

Don't Worry Be Happy: The Guide to Mood Therapy and Mood Cures

By: Eric Taffer

I0442128

PUBLISHERS NOTES

This publication is intended to provide helpful and informative material. It is not intended to diagnose, treat, cure, or prevent any health problem or condition, nor is intended to replace the advice of a physician. No action should be taken solely on the contents of this book. Always consult your physician or qualified health-care professional on any matters regarding your health and before adopting any suggestions in this book or drawing inferences from it.

The author and publisher specifically disclaim all responsibility for any liability, loss or risk, personal or otherwise, which is incurred as a consequence, directly or indirectly, from the use or application of any contents of this book.

Any and all product names referenced within this book are the trademark of their respective owners. None of these owners have sponsored, authorized, endorsed, or approved this book.

Always read all information provided by the manufacturers' product labels before using their products. The author and publisher are not responsible for claims made by manufacturers.

Trade Paperback Edition

Manufactured in the United States of America

WHAT YOU WILL LEARN IN THIS BOOK
How This Book Will Help You and Why

When someone suddenly becomes upset, it often does not make sense. One moment, the person is happy and carefree, and the next, they are moody, irritable and maybe even belligerent. While it may seem there should be no excuse for such mood swings, there are a variety of legitimate causes for this behavior. Although this type of behavior should never be encouraged, it is important that people have a thorough understanding of the causes of others' behavior and sometimes even their own!

This book was created to help you overcome mood swings and depression with revolutionary strategies using mood therapy techniques!

ABOUT THE AUTHOR

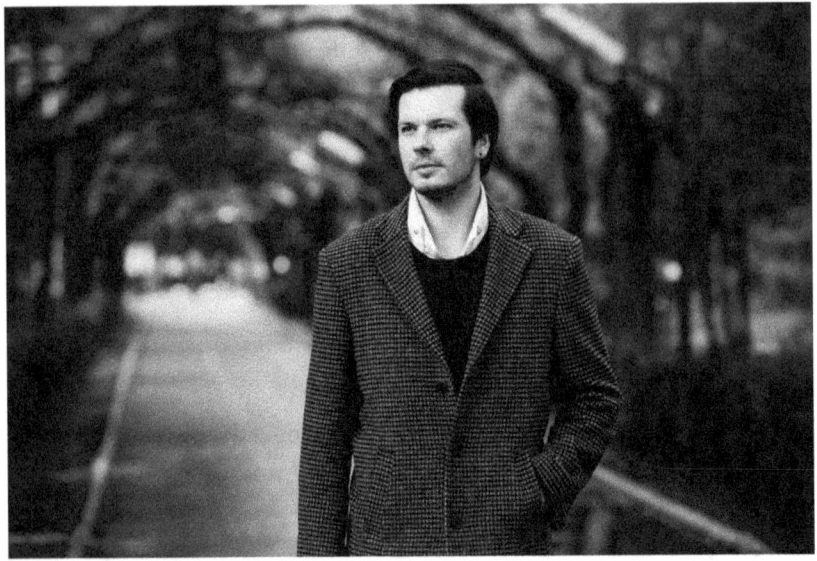

Eric Taffer grew up watching his mother struggle with mood problems. This problem got even worse after she had her last child, his little brother Michael. He vowed then to find viable solutions for persons with severe mood disorders. Through his initial research he was able to get his mother additional help and this led to a great improvement in her mood. He was then encouraged to share this knowledge with others so that they too may benefit from the alternate therapies that had worked for his mother.

Eric aims to inform and educate the reader. He has compiled all the information he had gotten from his research and put it all in one book which is easy to read and understand. He still lives in his hometown of Watertown, New York with his wife and two children. His mother is his greatest muse and research partner.

TABLE OF CONTENTS

How The Moods May Change Us All

"My best personality trait that I think I'm very approachable. And my worst is that I can be moody."

- Enrique Iglesias

CHAPTER 1- WHAT DOES IT REALLY MEAN TO BE MOODY

If you've ever been called moody and wonder what it meant then there are a number of things you should be aware of. People usually refer to someone as moody when they exhibit frequent erratic or displaced emotions like anger, sadness, or unwarranted paranoia.

A moody person can seem frightening to those around them because they seem to fly off the handle easily or act disinterested or mean when interacting. This state of emotional turmoil is thankfully temporary and situational in most cases, meaning that once the event that is making the person upset is over they can return to a normal, balanced state of mind. There are many reasons a person can act moody. Below are just a few.

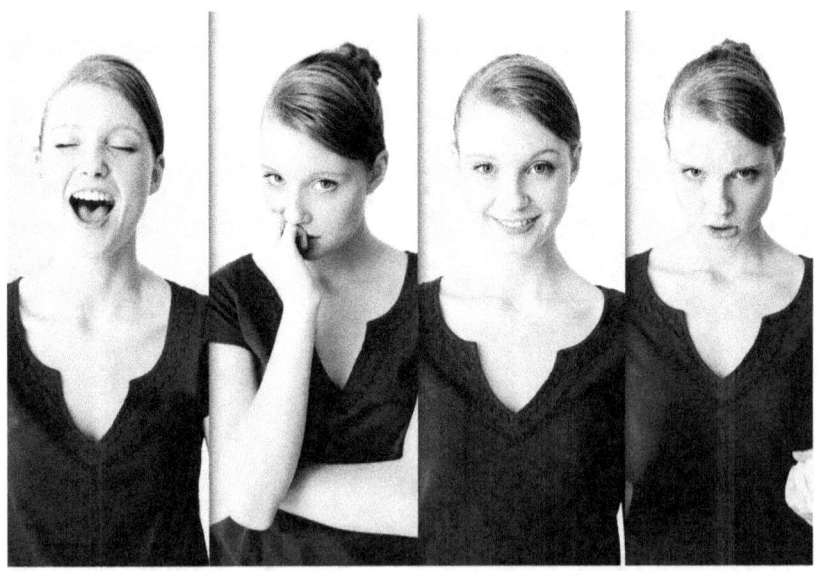

Personal Issues: Trouble at home, a death in the family, or work issues can make anyone feel anti-social or grumpy. When interacting with moody people remember that they are human too and may be experiencing personal difficulties that are causing them to feel alienated. If you feel that you yourself have become moody, then it is important to attempt to be considerate to those around you. Nothing is worse than taking something out on your friends in a mean spirited way, only to regret it later.

Depression Issues: Moodiness that becomes chronic, or frequent and long lasting, can point to deeper problems with depression or a chemical imbalance. If someone feels consistently isolated and sad for long enough without a break it can cause permanent malfunctions in the way they interact with the world. Depression can lead to more serious consequences like suicide and should be treated seriously.

Resentments: Resentment against people, situations, or loss can cause a person to become moody. The word resentment in Latin means, "To feel something over and over again." Resentment, if left unhealed, can cause someone to feel like they are being eaten alive by their own negative emotions.

Sometimes resentments simply build in a person's life to the point where they become permanently moody. If you have resentments it is important to try very hard to forgive and move on in order to be able to achieve true happiness. Resentment never hurts what it is directed towards; it only hurts the holder.

Justified Anger: Sometimes people act moody because they are not getting their needs met in some way or another, either emotionally or physically. In these cases it is very important to try to talk out what may be making the person feel defensive or upset. This can be done with a friend or a therapist. If functioning properly, emotions exist to guide us out of situations that have become toxic or no fun anymore. In these cases, negative emotions should be honored, the situation should be discussed by all parties, and hopefully grievances resolved.

In short, there are many reasons why a person can become moody or exist in a state of permanent moodiness. Problems can range from family or work related issues. People who are moody could be experiencing relationship trauma or financial burdens. A moody person could be plagued by deeper psychological problems, or simple have a grim world view developed by years of built up resentments.

Many education resources exist to help people out of their funk. Whether you are a moody person, or you are dealing with a moody person, the first step is to try to talk the issues out. If the problems go deeper than a friendly conversation will help, then it should be decided if further measures need to be taken such as talk therapy or medication. The other alternative is emotional anguish which doesn't seem like a good option.

CHAPTER 2- SO WHAT CAUSES MY MOOD SWINGS

When someone suddenly becomes upset, it often does not make sense, does it – so we know that they go from super cool to super agitated so one moment, the person is happy and carefree, and the next, they are moody and irritable. – What really causes it?

Some of the most common causes of mood swings occur only in women. For instance, it is not at all unusual for a woman to experience sudden sadness before she begins her monthly cycle. This is known as Premenstrual Syndrome, or PMS.

The moodiness will usually go away as soon as a woman starts her menstrual cycle. In addition, a woman is easily upset when she is pregnant due to the ***constant changing of estrogen levels*** in the body.

This can cause a woman to be extremely happy and extremely sad within a short period of time. The third common cause of moodiness unique only to women is menopause. (*We cover Post-Partum Depression later in this book*)

During this time, there is much less estrogen in the body, as the woman's body is experiencing difficult hormonal changes that will make her unable to reproduce. It is also not unusual for a woman to experience very low self-esteem during menopause.

Puberty is another cause associated with moodiness not only in females, but in males as well. When children begin the transition from childhood to adulthood, they gain something they did not have before; self-awareness. Children become very aware of their strengths and weaknesses at this time. Too often, they focus most on their weaknesses. As a result, they typically feel misunderstood and frustrated.

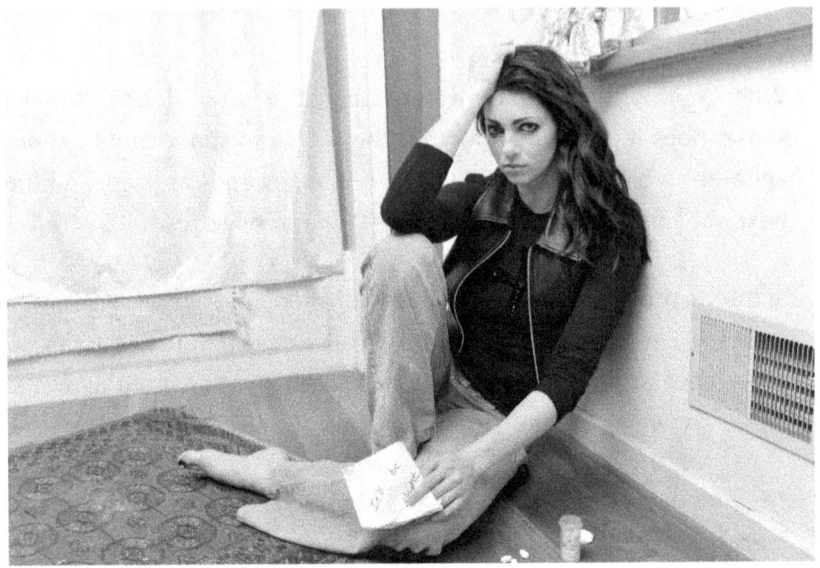

Also, there are <u>many psychological causes attributed to sudden mood changes</u>. These causes are sometimes the most overlooked, because many people see psychological disorders as an excuse to behave badly.

Though that is sometimes the case, it is more important to understand that psychological issues are sometimes the cause of mood swings in some people. Perhaps one of the most common disorders associated with moodiness is bipolar disorder.

One of the defining characteristics of this issue is when a person reacts negatively to a positive situation, and positively to a negative situation. When someone struggles with bipolar disorder, their next mood is truly unpredictable.

Depression is another psychological issue where people have extreme changes in mood. Depression is defined as an overall feeling of constant sadness that lasts for longer than two weeks. Many who are only temporarily sad use the term 'depression' so loosely and do not understand the psychological definition.

Those who really are depressed are extremely sad, extremely happy, and then extremely sad again. The cycle repeats itself many times. Aside from bipolar disorder and depression, there are many other psychological disorders that can cause mood swings.

A lot of people have health concerns. Because of these health concerns, many feel the need to regularly take medication.

Though medication is often a temporary solution to a problem, it is sometimes notorious for leaving horrible side effects on those who take it. While sudden mood swings are one of the least important side effects to be concerned about, they can still be a great problem.

Stress is a great cause of mood swings. It can be easy for a person to feel overwhelmed with everything going on in their life. People unrealistically attempt to juggle every aspect of their lives, but to no avail. As a result, these people usually experience great mood swings.

Indeed, mood swings can be extremely frustrating not only for the one experiencing it, but for the others around that person. However, it is significant that people do their best to sympathize with themselves and those around them. The problem cannot begin to be properly solved until the cause behind the problem is thoroughly understood.

CHAPTER 3- **DEPRESSION** THE MAIN FACTOR

The main type of treatment doctors prescribe for depression is medication. Most anti-depressant medication does have side effects. Doctors try to pick the medication that has a side effect that will help the patient. For example, if a patient's depression is causing them to not be able to sleep at night, then the doctor might prescribe an anti-depressant whose side effect is drowsiness.

On the other hand if someone is eating as a symptom of their depression, there are some medications that help control an appetite. In most circumstances, a physician will need to try different medications to find the one best suited to the patient.

They may also opt to combine some medications. The trouble with most anti-depressants is that if they are stopped abruptly, the symptoms can return but more severely. Always seek medical advice before stopping any anti-depressant.

The next alternative treatment for depression that doctors prescribe is psychotherapy. Psychotherapy or counseling is a treatment where you discuss your problems with a trained professional. They listen and counsel you on the best options for you to deal with your problems.

Most causes for depression are outside factors that the person doesn't feel like they are able to handle. Talking with someone can give an individual a perspective on their problems and the counseling to help deal with them. Doctors will typically recommend psychotherapy with medications. This combination is 80 - 90% effective in most depression cases.

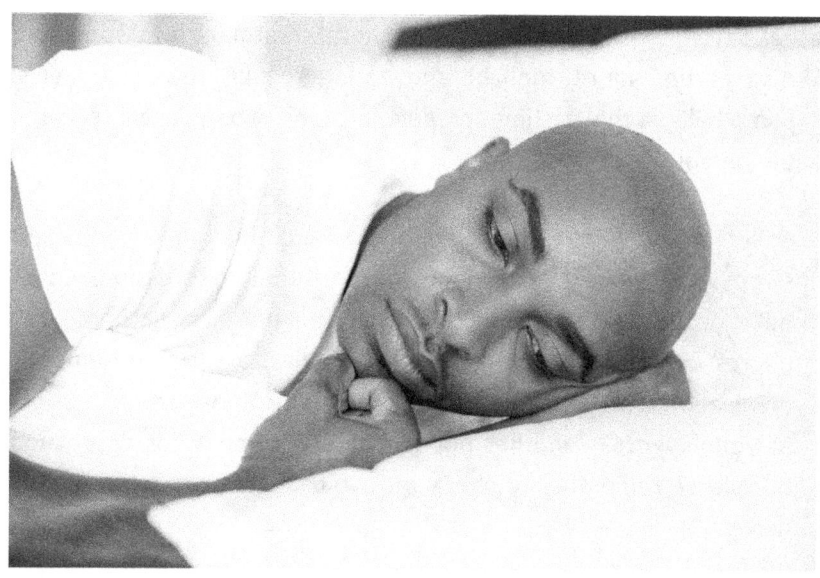

The third option doctors have to treat depression is electric shock therapy or ETC. This treatment is usually prescribed when medications and therapy have not worked.

The term electric shock therapy has a negative response in most people's mind. Current electric shock therapy is very different than it was 20 years ago. This was when people had electrodes attached to their heads and had electricity run through their bodies. This is the picture most people have when the term ETC is mentioned.

Today's methods are very different and effective. Patients of electric shock therapy are under anesthesia and typically done on an out-patient basis. The electric shock is only delivered to a small section of the brain. The recovery time is short and most patients have few side effects. Results of electric shock therapy are also more quickly seen for depression than that of medications or therapy.

Some people suffering from depression opt not to seek treatment with medical doctors but try more natural treatments. Massages to get better circulation is a popular natural treatment for depression. Also getting more sunlight and eating regular balanced meals. Some believe that fasting on apple juice for two days will recharge the nervous system.

Others believe that by avoiding caffeine and obtaining a good night sleep will help break someone out of their depression. Other believe that nasal drops of warm sesame oil will help with depression. Many believe that a regular exercise routine or medication will help reduce the stress that will lead to depression. St. John's wort is another popular natural remedy for depression but please remember to check with your doctor before taking any herbs.

Whether someone wishes to seek treatment through a medical provider or choose a natural remedy, the options for the treatment of depression is a personal decision based on the individual.

MEDICAL TREATMENT OF DEPRESSION – DOES IT REALLY WORK?

Antidepressants can be useful in treating those who suffer from moderate to severe depression and related disorders such as obsessive compulsive disorder and social anxiety disorder. There are many different options when it comes to moderate to severe depression treatment.

If one medication does not work, then it is possible that adding another or replacing it may alleviate some depression symptoms. Here is a list of some popular antidepressant medications.

FLUOXETINE

Uses

Sold under the brand name Prozac, this medication is part of a class of drugs known as the selective serotonin reuptake inhibitors (SSRIs).It works primarily by acting upon the brain chemical serotonin. It is also used to treat obsessive compulsive disorder, bulimia nervosa and panic disorder.

Side Effects

Fluoxetine may cause an allergic reaction in some people. Signs include skin rash, itchy eyes, difficulty breathing, or swelling of the mouth or throat. Other side effects of fluoxetine are sexual dysfunction, and a possible increased risk of suicidal thoughts in people age 25 and under.

BUPROPION

Uses

Known by the brand name Wellbutrin, this drug is considered atypical among antidepressants because it cannot be placed precisely within any of the other classes. It is thought that bupropion acts by affecting the reuptake of serotonin, norepinephrine and dopamine. Aside from its use as an antidepressant it's also frequently prescribed in lower doses as a smoking cessation aid under the brand name Zyban.

Side Effects

The most common side effects of this drug are headaches and insomnia. Unlike SSRIs, atypical antidepressants, like bupropion, do not generally cause sexual dysfunction.

DESIPRAMINE

Uses

Sold under the brand name Norpramin, desipramine is known as a tricyclic antidepressant (TCA) which is an older class of antidepressants. TCAs are generally not used as a first line of treatment due to their higher risk of side effects. They are more often used as an alternative or supplemental treatment in situations in which the patient is not showing adequate improvement with just SSRIs or SNRIs.

Side effects

Like other TCAs, desipramine has antimuscarinic effects such as dry mouth and nose, blurred vision and elevated body temperature, however the effects are less severe than with other TCAs. Other side effects include drowsiness, dizziness and sexual dysfunction.

PAROXETINE

Uses

Known by the brand name Paxil, this drug primarily affects serotonin reuptake and belongs to the selective serotonin reuptake inhibitor class of antidepressants. Aside from depression, paroxetine is also prescribed in a low dose form to treat post-traumatic stress disorder, social anxiety disorder and menopausal hot flashes.

Side Effects

Paroxetine, like other SSRIs, is known to cause sexual dysfunction. Some specific side effects include lack of interest in sex, inability to become aroused and difficulty reaching orgasm. These side effects are generally reversible, however, in some cases they become permanent. Other side effects of paroxetine could include nausea, diarrhea, dry mouth, insomnia and sexual dysfunction.

DULOXETINE

Uses

Known by the brand name Cymbalta, this drug belongs to a newer class of drugs known as serotonin-norepinephrine reuptake inhibitors (SNRIs). It is prescribed to treat major depressive disorder and generalized anxiety disorder as well as musculoskeletal pain and peripheral neuropathy.

Side Effects

The most commonly reported side effects of Duloxetine are dizziness, insomnia, dry mouth and drowsiness. Like other antidepressants, sexual dysfunction has been reported, however not as often as with selective serotonin reuptake inhibitors.

If an individual's depression is not improved by other treatment options, then prescription medication can be an effective answer. Since there are several different kinds of antidepressants and each one works in a slightly different way, one must work with their doctor to find the right medication or combination of medications that satisfactorily improves their depression symptoms.

CHAPTER 4- SO ARE YOU BIPOLAR, DEPRESSED OR JUST MOODY

The term **_"bipolar"_** tends to be thrown around loosely. Often it is used about any person who seems to have mood swings or a temper and it is often used as an insult. Real bipolar disorder, however, is no joke and needs to be diagnosed and managed with proper medication for the patients' well-being and safety.

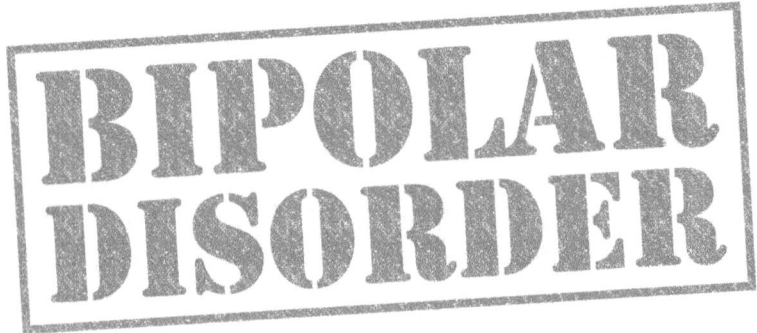

Typical markers can vary from case to case with some people experiencing euphoria, delusions and exhibiting very risky, impulsive behavior. Other markers are more subtle and can include a poor performance at work or in school as well as increased drive to achieve life goals.

Diagnosing bipolar disorder can be tricky. There are three levels of bipolar disorder, bipolar disorder I, bipolar disorder II and cyclothymic disorder.

Bipolar disorder I is severe and can be dangerous, as it often means engaging in risky behavior.

BIPOLAR II

Bipolar II is less severe and allows a person to lead a normal life, even though they may experience a significant amount of mood swings which can lower their quality of life. Cyclothymic disorder is the mildest form of bipolar disorder and often involves depression with less severe mood swings than the prior forms.

Living with an undiagnosed form of bipolar disorder can be extremely challenging for you and those around you. People may feel as if they are constantly walking on egg shells, waiting for a manic or depressive phase to appear.

The most severe cases of bipolar disorder can be physically dangerous as the patient can lose all common sense and engage in dangerous behavior such as walking on the high way, cooking with dangerous chemicals or wandering through a freezing cold winter storm with no clothing.

It can be extremely difficult to diagnose the disorder at this level as it shares common signs with paranoia and schizophrenia. If a child is under the care of a person suffering from this level of bipolar disorder it can be potentially harmful for the child, both mentally and physically.

The two other levels of bipolar disorder are less severe and can be somewhat easier to diagnose. In spite of this, even the lower levels of the disorder can prove to be difficult to live with. A person might also be less likely to seek help (or be forced to seek help) for the milder versions of the condition, as it can be hard to differentiate from other forms of depression.

As a result, many people who suffer from bipolar disorder are unaware of their condition and do not receive treatment. Treatment plans can be hard to work out as the medication given takes weeks to kick in and may have to be adjusted from person to person. Some of the heavier medications can cause an increase in weight or cause the patient to experience little emotion to the point that it can deprives them of their quality of life.

Because proper dosage is so important and varies from person to person, it is extremely important that the patient be monitored closely when starting or switching medications.

It is also worth mentioning that many bipolar patients tend to have an urge to get off the medication as soon as they feel "normal" which can send them spiraling back to a manic or depressive phase.

Dealing with bipolar disorder can be challenging for all parties involved. Proper treatment can tremendously improve the quality of life for both the patient and those around him. It may take some time to figure out the correct dosage for each individual but the result is well worth it and brings with it a much higher quality of life.

CHAPTER 5- CAN CBT BE USED TO HELP TREAT DEPRESSION?

Treating depression often requires multiple approaches. While some therapists take the natural and behavioral approaches, a number of therapists and physicians prescribe light medications to help an individual suffering from depression. In this modern age, depression can also be effectively treated with a successive approach, also known as cognitive behavioral therapy. This therapy is an effective treatment for depression, as per modern healthcare and science.

The goal of cognitive behavioral therapy is to help the individual in recognizing his pattern of thinking, negative behavior, and changes in his physical state. Once the person recognizes these, he or she can effectively work towards the healing process.

Cognitive behavioral therapy includes two different approaches. The first one is the base of the therapy, which focuses on the affected individual's moods and thoughts.

The second approach targets actions, behavioral patterns, and moods through the approach of behavioral therapy. In short, the first approach targets a person's thoughts, whereas the second therapy targets an individual's actions and behaviors.

This combined approach, then effectively helps the individual in managing stress and depression eventually by minimizing troubled thinking, negative behavior, and depressing thoughts.

Here is a brief overview about cognitive behavioral therapy.

How does this approach work?

Treating depression requires a collective approach than an individual one. Usually, therapists start with psychoanalysis and psychodynamic therapies. Such therapies often take years to treat depression effectively. However, cognitive behavioral therapy is a relatively short-term approach. As these therapies target specific areas, the entire approach usually takes only 10 to 20 individual sessions.

During each session, the therapist identifies and treats individual problems relevant to depression. Whether it is behavioral problem or negative thoughts that contribute to the patient's depression, the CBT therapist will analyze that first before taking a specific approach to treat depression. The therapist first identifies the current situation by analyzing the behavioral patterns of thinking.

Maintaining a journal:

Usually, CBT therapists ask patients to maintain a journal. This is to help the individual in maintaining record events, their thought patterns, and other signs of negative behavior. Therapists will give you a list of behavioral patterns and thought types so that you can easily recognize and make a note of these behavioral changes easily. This includes sudden thought changes, automatic negative reactions, personalization thoughts, mental pattern change with single negative thought, and disqualifying the positive experiences. Therapists insist on using the journal because therapists can work easily towards their healing process by recognizing their behavioral patterns.

Using a journal also helps each patient in learning self-control, avoiding sudden reaction, combating emotional behavior, and practicing self-talk. This will eventually help the person in reflecting on his behavioral pattern and cope with it appropriately. Patients can easily practice these methods on their own and learn to control their depression in an effective way.

Disorders treated by Cognitive behavioral therapy:

This treatment is widely used for treating depression and several other similar conditions in patients of all ages. Some of the disorders treated by this therapy include, anxiety disorder, panic attack, depression, binge eating behavior, anorexia, and bulimia, bipolar disorder, phobias, schizophrenia, sleep disorders, and substance abuse. Kids and adolescence with social behavioral problems are also treated by cognitive behavioral therapy.

Sometimes, your therapist will prescribe some medications for you to combine with the treatments of cognitive-behavioral therapy for best results.

Chapter 6- You Need To Take Care Of Your Emotional Health

Your emotional health is determined by how you feel about yourself and your life. It is very important to maintain a serene and calm mind and body in order to have good emotional health. People that are always on edge or paranoid do not have good emotional health. So how is emotional health different from mental health?

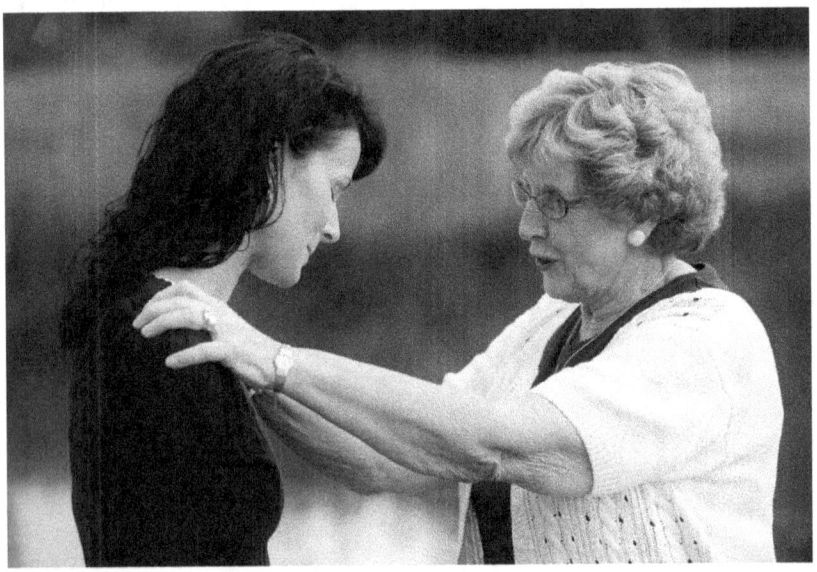

Mental health, physical health, and emotional health are like three screws holding up a heavy shelf. If one screw fails the other two, if strong, can compensate for a while and continue to hold the shelf in place. But, if steps aren't taken to replace that other screw, eventually the other two will weaken under the extra stress until the whole shelf is at risk.

Emotional, physical and mental health are not the same but are inter-related. What is good for one is likely good for all. One example is exercise. People who work out regularly talk about its centering effects on the mind and heart. Though it is most necessary for physical well-being, physical exercise can improve mental function and encourage emotional balance too. Likewise a person who finds love is apt to feel better physically and become more mentally centered than a person who is still out there searching.

Emotional health is most at risk during times of great upheaval. Divorce, moving, death of a loved one, retirement, these represent life changes that can be emotionally devastating. On the other hand, times of change also present great opportunities for emotional growth and personal transformation if we can reach past the stress and grief and find a healthier path to move forward.

At these times when your emotional health is most at risk, you need to take extra steps to care for your emotional self. One way to improve emotional health is to express what you are feeling in a positive way. Now is the time to start a journal or a blog. Take a painting class or write some poetry from the heart. Write a country or blues song.

Turn on some favorite music and dance your feelings out, but not just once. Try to express whatever you are feeling creatively, every day. Keeping it all bottled up inside until the inevitable eruption occurs is both self-destructive and socially irresponsible.

It is important to get negative things off your mind and heart if you want to continue to have mental and emotional sanity. Never let things that bother you in your life go unsettled with you feeling a heavy burden of guilt or sadness. Having a hobby or a good healthy social life will allow you to release built up tension you may have.

Another positive step you can take to become more emotionally healthy is to volunteer to help others. It may sound counter-intuitive to give of yourself when you are most in need. But, whether you cook at a soup kitchen or help clean at no-kill shelter, nothing will make you feel better emotionally than making other lives a little better. It also helps put our own circumstances in perspective when we look around at others who are hurting just as badly, if not more than we are.

Lastly, you need to do what you can to stay healthy physically and mentally during times of great emotional trauma. Eating right and getting enough sleep and exercise might not be easy but can work miracles for your emotional well-being.

Also consider seeing a therapist. If nothing else it is someone to talk to about your feeling who isn't directly involved in what has happened to you. Friends and family, are likely feeling their own emotional upset now, if only for the fact that they are worrying about you. Stay positive at all times and you will keep good emotional and mental health.

FIVE SIMPLE STEPS TO IMPROVE EMOTIONAL HEALTH AND BEAT MOODINESS

It is common practice for people to take vitamins to keep their physical bodies in shape. Consumers take calcium for healthy bones, B12 for energy, biotin for healthy skin and a host of other supplements to maintain physical wellness.

Humans constantly strive to improve physical health, but it is not as common for people to put the same time and effort into improving emotional health. Five things that can assist with improving emotional health are:

Meditation.

Five minutes of day of quiet reflection can help calm your mind. A calm mind is a healthy mind.

Regular exercise.

Exercising is not just for weight loss. When you exercise, your body releases endorphins. These endorphins increase happiness. This is a scientific fact. A thirty minute walk, a bike ride or simply dancing your heart out to a few of your favorite songs improve emotional health.

Be honest about your feelings to yourself.

It is completely acceptable to get upset about negative circumstances that occur, but it is not okay to dwell in those circumstances. For example, if a love one passes away, it is natural to grieve. It's natural to feel sadness, anger and despair at the loss. Give yourself time to feel those emotions and be honest about those feelings, but don't linger there. The truth is that you have no control over whether a person lives or dies, but you can control how you cope with the loss.

Think Happy, Grateful Thoughts.

Easy right? The difference between success and failure is perspective. Have you ever had a conversation with a friend who was upset about something, but every time you suggested a solution, he or she found some reason why the solution would not work? If you have never encountered that person, then it's highly likely that you are that person.

Don't be that person. Being happy is a choice. Write out a list of things for which you are grateful. Read this list every single day and add to it. Read it when you a feeling down. If you find that you have nothing to be grateful for, then you are choosing unhappiness in your life by not recognizing that virtually everyone can be grateful for something.

Talk to someone or write out your feelings.

Talking out issues and getting feelings off of your chest can drastically improve emotional health. Do not talk to just anyone. Do not talk to someone who is negative or critical. Do not talk to someone who will judge you or give you unsolicited advice. You know who those people are, so just don't do it.

The purpose for sharing your feelings is to simply share them without criticism and to organize the thoughts out loud. If you do not have anyone in your life who you can talk to without the fear of them passing judgment, then take the time to write your private thoughts down and think about changing your social circle.

Unfortunately limiting contact with family and certain friends can be the key to emotional wellness. If you have thoughts about hurting yourself or others in a serious way, then you should talk to a professional. These thoughts are not normal. If you think that your life it not worth living or you are so unimportant that you don't need to live, it simply is not true. There are free counselling services all over the country that can help you gain clarity.

Emotional well-being is just as important as physical well-being. Meditation, regular exercise, positivity, honesty and sharing with others are just a few steps that can be taken toward improving emotional health.

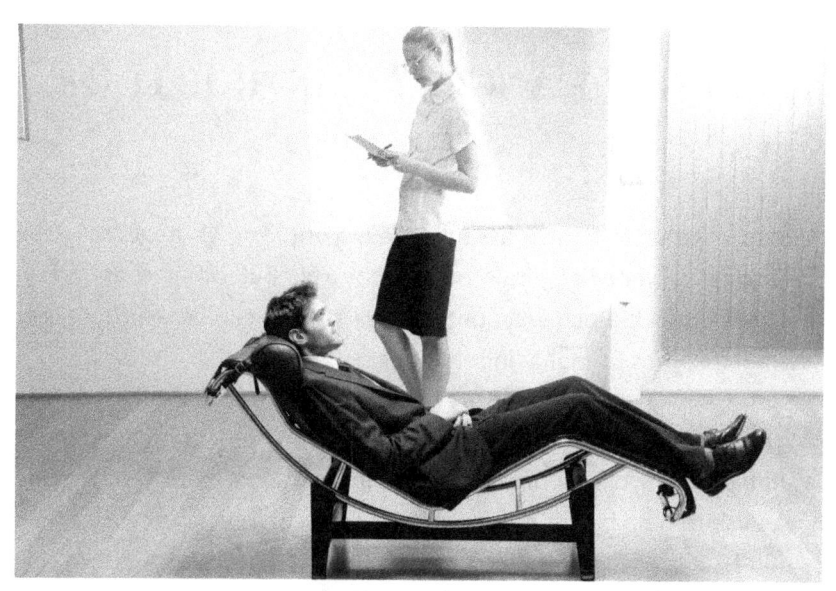

CHAPTER 7- ANGER? CONTROL IT OR ELSE

Road rage, bar fights, assault - everyone knows anger can be dangerous when it spirals out of control. But other than a few clichés - punch a pillow, count to ten - society can be weirdly silent when it comes to managing that anger.

While anyone having serious problems with anger management should seek professional help, here are five simple tips that anyone can use to help better manage their anger.

Identify and Avoid Your Anger Triggers

Simply put, an anger trigger is something that sets a person off, "triggering" their anger. These are different for everyone, and can range from engaging in high-stress situations such as driving in heavy traffic to waiting in line at the Post Office. Some anger triggers may be unavoidable, but others can be eliminated altogether by altering a daily routine or simply leaving a situation that seems likely to become an anger trigger.

Learn To Relax

"Just relax" is something people suffering from anger management issues may be sick of hearing. However, there are useful relaxation techniques that can be learned to help relax in anger-inducing situations that are difficult or impossible to avoid. The simplest of these is breathing deeply - not up in the chest area, but down from the diaphragm.

Slowly repeating a calming word or phrase like "relax" or "calm down" can also help. This is a technique that has been used to aid in meditation for centuries. Visualization can also help in a similar way; some people imagine a "happy place" such as a childhood haunt or an ideal vacation spot.

Reason With Yourself

When angry, people often speak in such absolutes as "this darn thing never works" or "this nonsense always happens." These exaggerated phrases, while often a symptom of the speaker's state of mind, can also reinforce that state of mind and create a feedback loop.

When using such language, it can be helpful to form the habit of stopping and examining the phrases and language used. If a person forces themselves to stop and remember that no, the copy machine doesn't really always break, only sometimes, that "emotional speed bump" can help slow things down and prevent runaway anger from spiraling out of control.

Find Humor and Laughter Anywhere

Humor can be a good way to ease tensions and release pent-up frustration. It can also invite sympathy from others better than uncontrolled rage. Jokes can also help an angry person see that their situation isn't as dire or important as they felt at first, giving them a chance to cool off and see things with a more reasonable perspective. However, be aware that using humor as a way to ignore anger and allow rage to fester unexamined can be unhealthy; anger should always be acknowledged, but humor can help channel it into less destructive directions.

Keep an Anger Diary

Reflection can often help identify sources of anger and unpack underlying issues that may be contributing to excessive anger. The benefit of keeping an "anger diary" is twofold: first, writing down thoughts and feelings while angry can serve as a healthy emotional release (venting), allowing anger to be safely expressed without potentially unhealthy suppression.

Second, an anger diary can also provide insight into the reasons behind the anger, which may help reveal a secondary source of anger or illustrate for the author the irrationality and unreasonableness of the anger.

These five techniques, while not a substitute for professionally-guided therapy, can help people with excessive anger to regain control. As with most behavioral issues, there's no "silver bullet" solution, so what works for some may not work for all.

CHAPTER 8- THE PETS HAVE IT

Many people are aware that pets can help improve one's own life but they aren't always sure why. In particular, pets help relieve stress and depression, which has been proven in a number of different studies.

The reasons vary but some of the main ways a pet can help reduce stress includes: responsibility, friendship/love, social support and mood elevation.

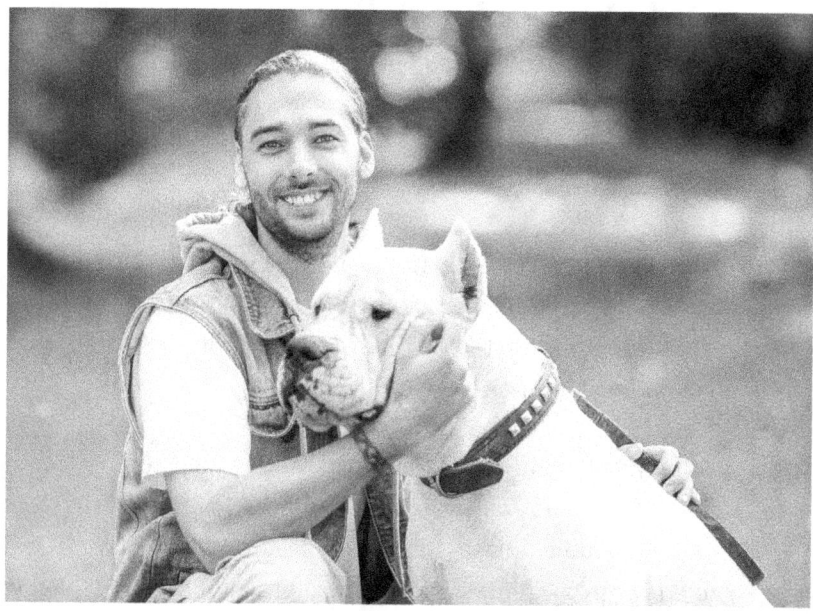

Animals do require a set amount of responsibility, which can be seen at first as a negative point because one can have stress over the care that pets require.

While it does take some financial and emotional expenditure in order to have a pet, these are minor aspects in comparison to how much the animals will give back in return. In fact, the slight addition of responsibility can help a person regain focus on their own life and needs.

They remind us that we need to take care of ourselves but in a non-judgmental, sometimes unconscious type of way. In fact, studies have shown that people often will exercise more, eat better and even sleep better when they have a pet than someone who does not.

Having a pet to take care of can increase one's own sense of value and show purpose for each day in a positive way.

Pet ownership also is known for creating a happier mood in many people. In fact, it doesn't even need to be owning a pet. Just having pictures of pets can increase many people's moods and there are many places online devoted to helping elevate moods through animals. Need writing encouragement?

One site allows the person to receive pictures of kittens and puppies after every 300 words written, or whatever word count and motivational image they would prefer but it all started with someone finding kitten pictures motivating.

And truthfully, it's hard to stay in a bad mood when coming home to a playful pet who will give unconditional love and affection. Which is why studies often show that anyone with pets are less likely to suffer from depression and negative mood issues. Having the animals provides support that helps cut away the stress of the day.

Which leads into the unconditional love and friendship aspect that pets provide their owners. Unlike dealing with human relationships and friendships, there is no worry about judgment or question of emotional return when it comes to pets.

They can alleviate the stress that social life provides because their attention doesn't have the same frustrations and requirements that others require. At the end of the day, the pet will be at home waiting.

Finally, they can help create social connections with other humans, even though they sometimes take the place of fixing the stress social situations can cause. Having a pet can push one towards social interaction and people like talking about pets. Comedians, authors, almost anyone is a potential social connection when pets are involved.

The slight nudge for social interaction is enough that it can help alleviate the negative energy that avoiding contact can create without having the situation become overbearing. Plus, after a social situation, one can always go home and receive the unconditional love that the pet provides no matter how the day went.

Overall, pet ownership will provide many benefits throughout a person's life and relieving stress is just one of the many attributes that they have to offer. Each animal has its own personality, quarks and level of companionship that it will provide.

There is a pet out there for almost anybody who wants to take up the joy that pets have to offer.

CHAPTER 9- EXPLAINING POSTPARTUM DEPRESSION

Having a baby can be an exciting time in a couple's life. There is the shopping for baby clothes, socks, and blankets. There is the fixing up the nursery. There is the keeping up with regular doctor's visits. But, having a baby can also be a stressful time; especially for a couple that is having their first child.

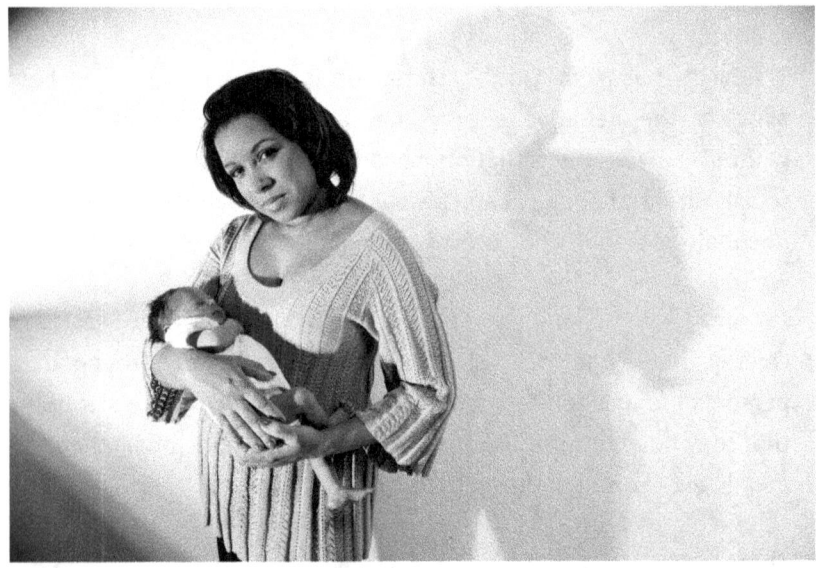

First time parents do not know what to expect. They often let their fantasies about parenthood run wild, thinking it is a walk in the park. It is a different story when the baby comes. The baby is constantly crying. He/she has to be fed, burp, and changed every four to six hours.

The new parents feel like their heads are going to explode. Having a baby can bring on postpartum depression.

Postpartum depression is a form of profound sadness that occurs soon after a baby is brought home from the hospital. It is brought on by the stress of caring for a newborn baby. Even though all parents with newborn babies can develop postpartum depression, new parents are the most susceptible to it.

The main reason is that they are inexperience. They are inexperienced with calming down an agitated baby. They are most likely to become quickly frustrated. Not having support from family and/or friends can worsen the situation. New parents without a support system are most likely to feel defeated, lash out, and abandon their parental responsibilities. Feeling like they have to abandon their crying baby for a few minutes make them more frustrated.

A heightened level of frustration will cause parents of newborns (in general) to display signs of PPD. They will out-of-the-blue begin crying, compulsively. They will not feel hungry enough to eat anything, even though they have not eaten all day.

They will not be able to get any sleep when their babies are asleep. And, they feel like horrible parents because they are taking five minute breaks.

Postpartum depression hinders them from doing the things that need to be done like cleaning, cooking, doing laundry, and tending to their babies. Fortunately for these parents, this form of depression is temporary. It lasts for a few weeks. There is, however, a form of PPD that can last much longer.

The type of postpartum depression that can last for months (or years) is known as postpartum depression psychosis. People that experience the psychotic form of PPD exhibit the same symptoms as people that do not experience this form of PPD. The only difference is that people in the second category occasionally experience hallucinations.

These hallucinations cause them to become paranoid. People that suffer from this type of PPD experienced traumatic events. They (women) have suffered a miscarriage, witnessed or experienced a heinous crime, or fought in a war. These people often dream about the events that traumatized them, sometimes behaving as if they are presently experiencing these traumas. It is wise for people that are experiencing postpartum depression in general to seek help.

Postpartum depression is not something that a person can overcome by himself/herself. Reaching out to love-ones is a great way to overcome it. PPD suffers that have frequent conversations with family and friends that lived their experience will better cope with the stresses of parenting newborn babies.

Exercising and getting a few naps in during the day while others babysit also helps. In the case of people that experience psychotic episodes, it is best for them to seek professional help. The best ways for them to overcome their PPD are with medication and counseling. The best way to overcome postpartum depression in general is with early detection.

Chapter 10- Parting Shots: How Not To Get Angry

Many of us will be, or already have been, in a heated argument with someone at least once in our lives. A lot of the time this will probably be with someone you are very close to. It is important to know how to handle yourself in a situation like this.

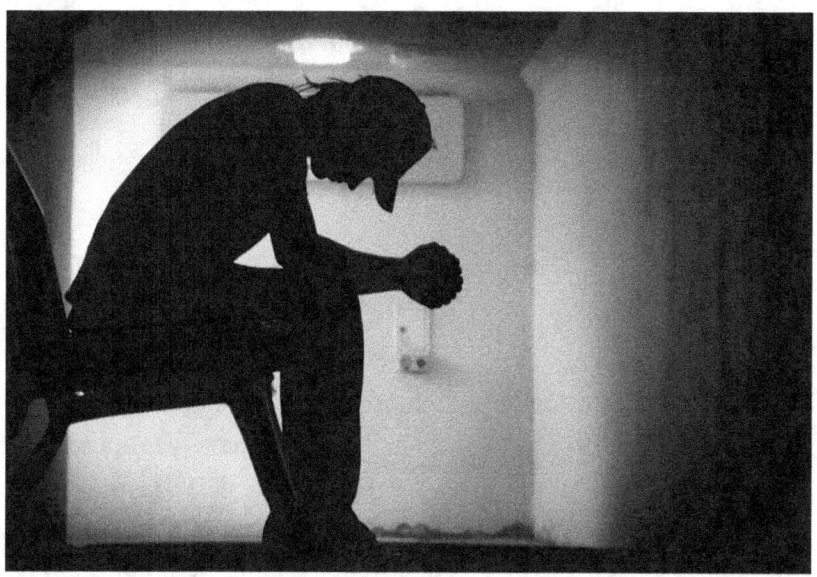

If you do not know how to calm yourself down in a heated argument, then things can escalate to something even much worse than they already are. In this article I will discuss 5 ways in which to calm yourself down when you are involved in a heated argument.

Work it out (exercise)

One good way to calm yourself down is to direct that anger or tension into a much more positive direction. Exercise is a great way to get some of that anger and aggression out from an argument.

You can do any type of exercise in order to calm yourself down. It really depends on the type of person you are. Running is one that I have found to be good for letting off some steam. There is also weight lifting or taking out some of your frustration on a heavy bag. It's really up to you.

Take deep breaths

This may seem like a bit of a cliché, and that is because it is. However, taking deep breaths is very effective at calming you down during and after a tense situation. It would also help to count while you are taking deep breaths as well. For example, count from one to twenty and then back down to one. This gives you something to focus your mind on other than what you were just arguing about.

Talk it out

Now, I do not mean try to talk it out with whoever you may have been arguing with, but talk to someone else instead. Talk to someone who you are close to and will not judge you, because a judgmental person will probably just make matters worse. You should try to talk to a close friend or a family member. Someone who always seems to be a good listener is a mother. Moms always seem to know the right thing to say in any situation. But any close friend or relative will do.

Walk it out

Sometimes just taking a long walk is just what the doctor ordered when you are involved in a heated a heated situation. Take a walk and try to think about what happened and what caused things to get so out of hand. A lot of the times once you come back from your walk, you are more level headed and maybe you will be able to talk things over in a more rational and civilized way.

Just let it go

This may seem a lot easier said than done. This is because it is a lot easier said than done. It takes a lot to be the bigger person and just let something go. Sometimes you may have to just swallow your pride and let whatever was bothering you go. Now, if you do not believe that you were at fault for the argument, then this may more difficult for you. However, in any argument, someone has to be the bigger person and let it go or it will never be resolved.

Arguments happen is just about every type of relationship, not matter how good the relationship is. Dealing with an argument without letting it get the best of those involved is the hardest part.

www.ingramcontent.com/pod-product-compliance
Lightning Source LLC
Chambersburg PA
CBHW070131290526
45789CB00005B/2199